Percutaneous Transluminal Coronary Angioplasty

*A Report of the National Confidential Enquiry
into Perioperative Deaths*

Data collection period
1 September 1998 to 31 August 1999

Compiled by:

K G Callum MS FRCS

F Whimster MHM

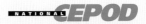

Published 21 November 2000 by the National Confidential Enquiry into Perioperative Deaths

35-43 Lincoln's Inn Fields, London WC2A 3PN
Tel: (020) 7831 6430
Fax: (020) 7430 2958
Email: info@ncepod.org.uk
Website: www.ncepod.org.uk

Requests for further information should be addressed to the Chief Executive

ISBN   0 9522069 9 4

A company limited by guarantee   Company number 3019382
Registered charity number 1075588

This report is printed on paper produced from wood pulp originating from managed sustainable plantations and is chlorine-free, acid-free, recyclable and biodegradable.

Additional information

This report is available for downloading from the NCEPOD website at www.ncepod.org.uk

Copies can also be purchased from the NCEPOD office.

The analysis of data from questionnaires is not included in full in this report.
A supplement containing additional data, and copies of the questionnaires,
is available free of charge from the NCEPOD office.

 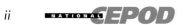

ACKNOWLEDGEMENTS

This report could not have been achieved without the support and cooperation of a wide range of individuals and organisations. Our particular thanks go to the following:

- The Royal College of Physicians and British Cardiovascular Intervention Society for supporting the concept of this study.

- The Local Reporters, whose names are listed in Appendix D.

- All those cardiologists whose names are listed in Appendix E, together with a small number of anaesthetists and surgeons, who contributed to the Enquiry by completing questionnaires.

- The Advisors whose names are listed overleaf.

- Those bodies, whose names are listed in Appendix B, who provide the funding to cover the cost of the Enquiry, together with the Department of Health who provided additional support.

- Mr Chris Macklin, Surgical Registrar, Derbyshire Royal Infirmary, for the illustrations on the front cover.

- Professor Tom Treasure for the drawing in Figure 6.

The Steering Group, Clinical Coordinators and Chief Executive would also like to record their appreciation of the hard work and tolerance of the NCEPOD administrative staff: Peter Allison, Fatima Chowdhury, Paul Coote, Sheree Cornwall, Jennifer Drummond and Dolores Jarman.

The views expressed in this publication are those of NCEPOD and not necessarily those of the National Institute for Clinical Excellence, or any other funding body.

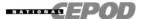

CLINICAL CONTRIBUTORS

NCEPOD COORDINATORS

K G Callum   Clinical Coordinator, NCEPOD and
Consultant General and
Vascular Surgeon,
Derbyshire Royal Infirmary

K M Sherry   Clinical Coordinator, NCEPOD and
Consultant Anaesthetist,
Northern General
Hospital NHS Trust, Sheffield

SPECIALTY ADVISORS

Anaesthesia

D K Whitaker   Manchester Royal Infirmary

Cardiology

M de Belder   South Cleveland Hospital

H H Gray   Southampton University Hospital
and Royal College of Physicians'
representative on
NCEPOD Steering Group

L D R Smith   Royal Devon and Exeter Hospital

Cardiothoracic surgery

T Treasure   St George's Hospital, London

G Venn   St Thomas' Hospital, London

CONTENTS

NATIONAL CEPOD

TABLES, FIGURES AND QUESTIONS

FOREWORD

We were delighted when those in the profession involved in this important modern development in treatment were prepared to contribute so enthusiastically to this NCEPOD survey. The consultants involved were not previously experienced in NCEPOD investigations and they have responded enthusiastically with a dramatically high rate of return. It was well recognised that as a specialty their data had been collected centrally and the results shown in the NCEPOD survey closely tally with the outcome of their own specialty audit.

Another important feature of this study is that it is one of the first times we have been able to gather reliable denominator data. This significantly affects the interpretation of the overall returns and hence enhances the importance of the report.

The cases reviewed in this survey were all severely ill patients and the outcome of interventions, only very recently deemed inappropriate, is impressive. The mortality rate is low and, as demonstrated by the report, consistent with the severity of illness of the patients under investigation.

This is a small survey by NCEPOD standards, but one of great importance, and demonstrates the value of the acquisition of reliable data by clinicians involved, and the importance of recording this on a national level to assess the quality of outcomes.

John Ll Williams
Chairman

SELECTED KEY POINTS

- Co-operation by participating hospitals was commendably high, with 98% of monthly returns being received (page 2).
- This is one of the first NCEPOD studies in which denominator data were collected (page 2).
- The overall mortality reported in this study is almost identical to that previously reported independently in surveys undertaken by the British Cardiovascular Intervention Society (BCIS) (page 3).
- There was very high consultant involvement in both the decision to undertake, and the performance of, PTCA procedures (pages 8 and 16).
- Operators were fully trained and considered to be suitably experienced to perform the procedure in almost all cases (page 16).
- The majority of cardiologists (95%) are complying with the BCIS recommendations on the number of procedures which should be performed each year (page 17).
- The majority of procedures in those patients who died were performed as an emergency in high risk patients with acute coronary syndromes (acute myocardial infarction or unstable angina) (pages 9-10).
- PTCA is very safe when performed as a planned procedure for patients with stable angina (page 9).
- A high proportion of patients had coexisting medical conditions (page 10).
- A high proportion of patients had moderate or severe left ventricular dysfunction and extensive coronary artery disease (pages 11-12).
- Intracoronary stents were inserted in approximately 50% of cases (page 15).
- Nearly half the patients were referred from another hospital (page 6).
- Some instances of delay in interhospital transfer were cited, but no patient was recorded as having deteriorated during the journey (page 6).
- Intra-aortic balloon pumps would appear to be under-used considering the fairly high proportion of patients reported to be in cardiogenic shock (pages 15 and 24).
- Very few patients underwent emergency or urgent CABG following PTCA (page 22).
- A designated recovery area was available in 81% of cases (page 23).
- There appears to be an under-use of glycoprotein IIb/IIIa receptor blockers in high risk PTCA (page 20).
- Ninety-four percent of catheter laboratory staff receive regular resuscitation training (page 18).
- The decision whether or not cardiopulmonary resuscitation (CPR) should be performed was made in a responsible way by experienced cardiologists (page 25).
- In 92% of cases the interventional centre held regular audit meetings (page 27).

 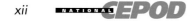

RECOMMENDATIONS

- Interventional cardiology centres should have a sufficient number of appropriately experienced clinicians and other staff to run an emergency PTCA service (pages 16-18).
- It is essential that there is an efficient system for transferring patients from the district general hospital to the interventional centre; ambulance services should be able to respond rapidly to calls for urgent transfer of patients requiring PTCA in the setting of acute myocardial infarction (pages 6-7).
- There is a need for consistency in the definition of cardiogenic shock, in order to give an accurate prognosis and compare outcomes of treatment (page 13).
- All catheter laboratory staff should have regular resuscitation training (page 18).
- Intra-aortic balloon pumps should be available for appropriate patients; staff should be familiar with their use (pages 15 and 24).
- Catheter laboratories should have a designated person responsible for checking that all necessary equipment is both present and functional (page 18).
- All catheter laboratories should have appropriately equipped recovery areas (page 23).
- Monitoring with pulse oximetry should be available for all cases and performed whenever sedation or opiates are used or oxygen therapy is required; this should be performed by an appropriately trained nurse or technician (page 18-19).
- Glycoprotein IIb/IIIa receptor blockers should be used more widely for patients undergoing high risk PTCA. Heparin doses should be adjusted accordingly, and monitored using activated clotting time (ACT) or equivalent, in order to minimise the risk of bleeding (page 20).
- Clinicians should be informed of the date and time that postmortem examinations are being performed and should do their best to attend; a copy of the postmortem report should always be sent to the appropriate clinician (pages 26-27).
- Regular audit meetings should be held in all interventional cardiology centres (page 27).
- For the practice of angioplasty and the assessment of its risk to be improved, and for patient consent to be better informed, comprehensive systems for recording patient and procedural data need to be in place. Data should be regularly audited and submitted to allow comparison with national averages (page 13).
- Hospitals should provide access to case records for audit purposes (page 27).

PERCUTANEOUS TRANSLUMINAL CORONARY ANGIOPLASTY (PTCA)

INTRODUCTION

Percutaneous transluminal coronary angioplasty (PTCA) has developed over the last twenty years. The basic principle is to introduce a guidewire and catheter via a needle in a peripheral artery, most commonly the femoral, and steer them round, under X-ray guidance, to the coronary arteries. A variety of devices may be used, most commonly a balloon catheter, to stretch a narrow area or block, restoring a channel for the blood to flow through (balloon angioplasty).

Other devices can be inserted into a diseased artery in a similar way. The most frequently used is a stent, a metal device which is mounted collapsed on a deflated balloon catheter; its structure is such that once expanded it will not collapse but keeps the artery open. Studies have shown that the artery is less likely to develop a further narrowing (restenosis) with a metal stent than with a balloon angioplasty alone[1, 2, 3]. Another advantage is that if the lining of the artery is disrupted by the balloon being expanded and starts to fold inwards (dissection) a stent may be used to hold it back and thus prevent the artery from becoming blocked. Approximately half the procedures in this report involved the use of stents.

Until relatively recently PTCA was used for patients with a single coronary stenosis who were in a stable condition. However, because of technical advances and increasing expertise, multiple coronary lesions, including occlusions, are now routinely treated with generally very good results[1,4]. In addition, patients with acute myocardial infarction (MI) may be treated as emergencies[5], including those who are extremely ill with severe heart failure. A high proportion of patients in this report (over 80%) had their coronary intervention performed as an emergency.

New drugs to prevent thrombosis have been developed (the IIb/IIIa antagonists) which are powerful antiplatelet agents, and these have been shown to reduce the likelihood of the artery occluding due to a blood clot[6,7,8]. When the patient's heart contraction is severely impaired, an intra-aortic balloon pump (IABP) may be used to support the circulation during and after an angioplasty procedure[9,10]. This is inserted into the aorta and connected to an external pump which is triggered by the electrocardiogram (ECG) so that its inflation and deflation are synchronised with the heart. Thus it is able to augment the failing heart while other measures are taken to improve its function.

DATA COLLECTION

Data was requested from all NHS hospitals undertaking PTCA procedures in England, Scotland, Wales and Northern Ireland, together with relevant hospitals in the independent sector. Participation was voluntary and a few hospitals chose, for a variety of reasons, not to participate.

Information on the total number of patients undergoing PTCA on a monthly basis, together with notification of any deaths occurring within 30 days of the procedure, were collected for the period 1 September 1998 - 31 August 1999.

Further details on the data collection and review process are given in Appendix C.

GENERAL DATA

Key Points

- *Co-operation by participating hospitals was commendably high, with 98% of monthly returns being received.*
- *This is one of the first NCEPOD studies in which denominator data were collected.*

MONTHLY RETURNS

Forty-six hospitals initially agreed to participate in the study, although five of these then failed to send in any monthly returns, reducing the number of participating centres to 41. Each hospital was required to send in a monthly return of all patients undergoing PTCA in the hospital. A total of 484/492 (98%) monthly returns were received.

A regional breakdown of the number of these monthly returns received is given in Table 1. The rate was commendably high (98%); only North Thames, Northern Ireland and Scotland failed to achieve a 100% return rate.

Table 1: Monthly returns by region				
Region	Number of participating hospitals	Monthly forms received	Monthly forms expected	Return rate
Anglia & Oxford	2	24	24	100%
North Thames	5	58	60	97%
North West	4	48	48	100%
Northern & Yorkshire	4	48	48	100%
South & West	3	36	36	100%
South Thames	3	36	36	100%
Trent	3	36	36	100%
West Midlands	3	36	36	100%
Wales	2	24	24	100%
Northern Ireland	2	23	24	96%
Scotland	5	55	60	92%
Independent sector	5	60	60	100%
Total	41	484	492	98%

REPORTED PROCEDURES

This is one of the first studies where NCEPOD has been able to collect data on the total number of procedures performed, as well as details of those patients who died. A total of 21 222 of these procedures were reported by the 41 participating hospitals in the year from 1 September 1998 to 31 August 1999, giving a mean of 518 procedures per centre.

REPORTED DEATHS

Key Points

- *The overall mortality reported in this study is almost identical to that previously reported independently in surveys undertaken by the British Cardiovascular Intervention Society (BCIS).*

- *Those patients who died following PTCA generally did so within the first few days of the procedure.*

Figure 1 shows that a total of 164 reports of deaths within 30 days of a procedure were received from the 41 participating centres, reducing to 157 when seven inappropriate reports were excluded (Table 2). A further five reports were received after the deadline of 29 February 2000 and one remained incomplete despite all efforts to identify missing information, leaving 151 cases for inclusion in the study.

In order to try to determine as accurate an estimate of mortality as possible only those centres that had a 100% return rate of monthly forms throughout the year, together with reporting at least one death, were included. Twenty-nine centres undertook 16 269 procedures in the year and reported 141 deaths, giving a mortality rate of 0.87%, almost identical to that reported independently by BCIS (0.91%) for the calendar year 1997[11].

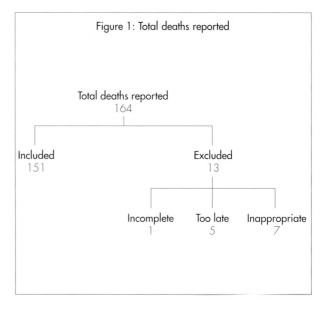

Figure 1: Total deaths reported

Total deaths reported
164

Included
151

Excluded
13

Incomplete
1

Too late
5

Inappropriate
7

Table 2: Inappropriate reports received and excluded	
Reason for exclusion	Number
More than 30 days *(day of procedure to day of death)*	2
Death outside study period	5
Total	7

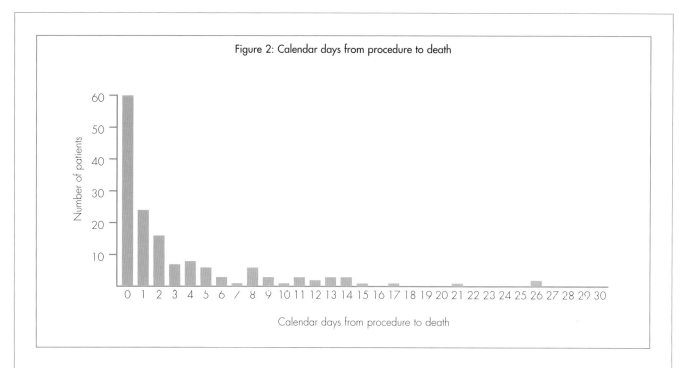

Figure 2: Calendar days from procedure to death

Figure 2 shows that half the deaths occurred in the first 24 hours and the majority of the remainder in the next few days. Figure 3 shows the distribution of age and sex.

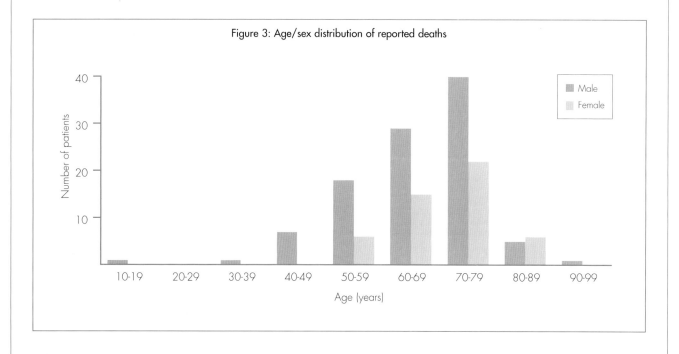

Figure 3: Age/sex distribution of reported deaths

Coronary artery disease is more common in men than women and hence it was expected that many more deaths would be reported for males. However, coronary artery disease in women may be under-diagnosed. The total number of procedures performed was not broken down by sex; without this more comprehensive data it is not possible to comment on whether there was any difference in the mortality rate between the sexes.

The one patient aged less than 20 years was a 17-year-old who had previously had several operations for congenital heart disease; he had a PTCA and stent for a fibrous stenosis of an aberrant coronary artery.

DISTRIBUTION AND RETURN OF QUESTIONNAIRES

Questionnaires were sent to the consultant cardiologist responsible for the care of each of the 151 patients included. Figure 4 shows the return and analysis rates of these questionnaires.

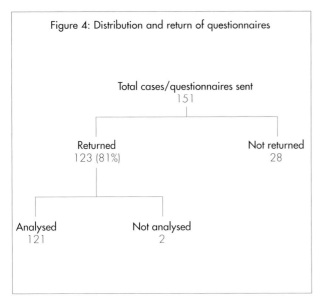

Figure 4: Distribution and return of questionnaires

Total cases/questionnaires sent
151

Returned
123 (81%)

Not returned
28

Analysed
121

Not analysed
2

Two questionnaires were incomplete and therefore excluded from further analysis.

In 27 cases where a questionnaire was not returned, no reason was offered for an inability to do so. In the remaining case the cardiologist indicated that the medical records could not be traced.

If an anaesthetist was involved in the care of the patient, a questionnaire was also sent to the relevant consultant. If the patient underwent CABG surgery subsequent to PTCA and before death, a further questionnaire was sent to the consultant cardiothoracic surgeon. Table 3 shows the distribution, return and analysis rates for all three types of questionnaire, by region.

The majority of regions are to be congratulated on their participation in this study, with most achieving return rates for cardiology questionnaires in excess of 80%; the relatively low return rates from North Thames (61%) and West Midlands (60%) are disappointing and it is unfortunate that the only questionnaire sent in relation to a case performed in the independent sector was not returned. The total number of questionnaires sent to anaesthetists (10) and surgeons (9) was small; nonetheless, it is disappointing that only five were returned from each, and that North Thames, again, had a particularly poor record, failing to return two out of three anaesthetic questionnaires, and neither of two surgical questionnaires.

Table 3: Regional distribution, return and analysis rates									
CQ = Cardiology questionnaire AQ = Anaesthetic questionnaire SQ = Surgical questionnaire	Questionnaires distributed			Return rate			Questionnaires analysed		
	CQ	AQ	SQ	CQ	AQ	SQ	CQ	AQ	SQ
Anglia & Oxford	3	1	1	100%	100%	100%	3	1	1
North Thames	23	3	2	61%	33%	0	14	1	0
North West	14	2	2	93%	50%	100%	13	1	2
Northern & Yorkshire	36	0	0	97%	-	-	34	0	0
South & West	4	0	0	100%	-	-	4	0	0
South Thames	21	0	1	81%	-	0	16	0	0
Trent	12	1	1	83%	100%	100%	10	1	1
West Midlands	15	0	0	60%	-	-	9	0	0
Wales	7	2	2	100%	50%	50%	7	1	1
Northern Ireland	0	0	0	-	-	-	0	0	0
Scotland	15	1	0	73%	0	-	11	0	0
Independent sector	1	0	0	0	-	-	0	0	0
Total	151	10	9	71%	56%	50%	121	5	5

CLINICAL DATA

The report hereafter deals only with those patients who died. Although we know the total number of procedures performed, we only have detailed information on those who died and for whom a questionnaire was completed and returned. The questionnaire was designed to follow the patient through from the initial referral and assessment, to the angioplasty and related aspects, and finally the care following the procedure.

REFERRAL PATHWAY

Source of angiogram

Table 4: Source of angiogram	
Hospital where angiogram performed	**Number**
The hospital undertaking the PTCA procedure	108
Another hospital	11
Not answered	2
Total	**121**

Table 4 shows that 9% (11/121) of the initial diagnostic angiograms were performed in hospitals not routinely undertaking angioplasty, with subsequent referral to an interventional centre being required. In the UK a large number of diagnostic angiograms are performed in district general hospitals not undertaking coronary angioplasty. At first sight, therefore, it might seem strange that only 9% of patients who died after subsequent angioplasty had their diagnostic angiogram performed outside the interventional centre. The likely explanation is that the majority of patients who died were very sick before the PTCA procedure, due to an acute MI. In these circumstances angiography would be undertaken immediately before the angioplasty procedure in the interventional centre.

Admission pathway

Key Points

- *Nearly half the patients were referred from another hospital.*

- *Some instances of delay in interhospital transfer were cited, although no patient in this study was recorded as having deteriorated during the journey.*

- *It is essential that there is a smooth and efficient system for transferring patients from the district general hospital to the interventional cardiology centre; ambulance services need to be made aware of the need for urgent transfer of patients in the context of myocardial infarction.*

- *About a quarter of patients were admitted via the A&E Department.*

Table 5 summarises from whence the patients came for their coronary angioplasty.

Table 5: Admission pathway	
Admission pathway	**Number**
From home (routine waiting list)	12
From home (urgent waiting list)	15
From another hospital	55
From A&E	33
From another ward in your hospital	6
Total	**121**

A recent report has confirmed that interhospital transfer for primary PTCA in high risk patients with acute myocardial infarction is safe and feasible within a reasonable period of time, and that short and medium term outcome is favourable[12]. Optimising the decision process and transport logistics may further improve outcome by reducing the total time of ischaemia.

A total of 55 patients were transferred from another hospital for their coronary intervention. In 41 of these cases the patient's condition deteriorated and in 34 of these this was before the transfer, and indeed this deterioration may have caused the need for transfer. In the remaining seven this deterioration occurred in the hospital where the procedure was performed, but prior to it being carried out. It is interesting to note that none was thought to have deteriorated during the actual journey. In the emergency situation once the decision has been made to proceed it is obviously important to do so without delay. There were deficiencies in the transfer facilities in four cases:

CASE 1 • *A 60-year-old patient with cardiogenic shock was delayed for four hours at the referring hospital for reasons that were not clear.*

CASE 2 • *An 80-year-old patient had a delay in the diagnosis of 'failed thrombolysis'. It was initially thought she had reperfused but on later review of the ECGs she had probably not reperfused at any stage, and was thus seven hours into the infarct when she was transferred for 'salvage angioplasty'.*

CASE 3 • *A 70-year-old patient was transferred by ambulance for a journey that normally took 20 minutes. On this occasion it took one hour and 20 minutes; no reason was given.*

CASE 4 • *The ambulance journey for a 52-year-old patient took two hours, instead of the usual 40 minutes; no reason was given.*

It is surprising that no deterioration during the transfer was recorded in the two patients who underwent prolonged journeys. If the transfer system is going to work there has to be an efficient and smooth method of transport. Although ambulance services have protocols for response times after emergency calls from outside hospital, there are no legal obligations for rapid transfer from one hospital to another. They do not appear to be aware of the need for urgent transfer of patients in acute myocardial infarction. It was the unanimous view of the advisors that this matter should be addressed.

Admission details

Type of ward

Details as to where the patient was first admitted at the interventional cardiology centre are given in Table 6. The majority (74%) were admitted either to the coronary care unit (CCU) or to a cardiac ward and only 16/121 (13%) patients went direct to the catheter laboratory. This reflects the preponderance of patients with myocardial infarction, whose admission would normally be to a CCU.

Table 6: Destination on admission	
Destination	Number
Coronary care unit (CCU)	63
High dependency unit (HDU)	4
Intensive care unit (ICU)	2
Cardiac ward	26
General medical ward	5
Direct to catheter laboratory	16
Other	2
Not answered	3
Total	121

Admitting consultant

Table 7: Admitting consultant	
Specialty	Number
Cardiologist	91
General physician	26
Cardiac surgeon	1
Other	2
Not answered	1
Total	121

The fact that the admitting consultant was a general physician in 26/121 (21%) cases reflects the high number of patients who were admitted as emergencies with acute coronary syndrome and the arrangement in many hospitals whereby acute cardiac patients are initially admitted under the care of whichever physician is on emergency take that day.

Decision making

Key Points

• *The decision to proceed with a PTCA was made by a consultant in almost all cases.*

• *A protocol giving guidance as to who should be referred for PTCA may be of help.*

Table 8 summarises who was responsible for making the decision to carry out the coronary intervention. This shows that there was a very high consultant input in the decision to proceed with angioplasty.

Delays before the PTCA

There was thought to be a medically inappropriate delay before the PTCA procedure was undertaken in six cases (5%). Two patients initially declined PTCA, but changed their minds when their condition worsened:

CASE 5 • *A 75-year-old patient was admitted with an acute MI in cardiogenic shock. For three hours she was unable to decide whether or not to proceed with the angioplasty.*

CASE 6 • *A 65-year-old patient initially declined PTCA but four hours later, when his condition had deteriorated, he agreed.*

Other than carefully and patiently explaining the situation, there is not much more one can do under these circumstances.

In a further two cases there was difficulty making the diagnosis or deciding when to change management:

CASE 7 • *A 66-year-old patient was admitted under the care of the general surgeons with epigastric pain. By the next morning the correct diagnosis of MI was made and the patient transferred to the cardiologist.*

CASE 8 • *A 68-year-old patient with a long history of ischaemic heart disease (IHD) and myocardial infarction dating back to 1981, and a further MI two months earlier, was admitted with further chest pain and ventricular tachycardia (VT). This was initially treated with amiodarone, but because of recurrent bouts of VT, cardioversion was performed. During this the patient had an asystolic arrest requiring cardiopulmonary resuscitation (CPR) and adrenaline. Following this he developed temporary heart block necessitating pacing, and he subsequently reverted to sinus rhythm. Finally, after six days, he was transferred to the cardiology unit.*

Table 8: Decision to perform the coronary angioplasty (121 cases; answers may be multiple)	
Decision maker	Number
Consultant interventionist undertaking procedure	99
Consultant cardiologist	23
Specialist registrar in cardiology	4

The cardiology advisors thought that earlier referral for revascularisation might have helped. Is this a situation where a protocol giving guidance as to who should be referred for PTCA may be of help?

There were two further cases where no reason was given for the delay.

PATIENT DETAILS AND RISK ASSESSMENT

This section reviews the admission category and degree of urgency, coexisting medical conditions, the degree of myocardial ischaemia and the extent of the patients' coronary artery disease. These are all factors which might influence the outcome following coronary angioplasty.

Admission category and urgency

Key Points

- *The majority of procedures in those patients who died were performed as an emergency in high risk patients.*
- *PTCA is very safe when performed as a planned procedure for patients with stable angina.*

The urgency of the PTCA was defined as follows:

Elective – A procedure performed at a time to suit both the patient and the operator.

Scheduled – An early procedure, but not immediately necessary, which includes routine follow-on PTCA after diagnostic angiography.

Emergency – A procedure required at the earliest possible opportunity.

Emergency (catheter complication) – As above, but following a complication of diagnostic angiography.

Table 9 shows that only 17% (21/121) of patients had the PTCA done as an elective or scheduled procedure, and that 99 (82%) had the procedure done as an emergency. The majority of the PTCAs performed throughout the country are done electively. There were very few deaths among the elective group in this study, which indicates the safety of PTCA when done as a planned procedure, confirming the findings of previous audits[4, 11].

Table 9: Urgency of the final procedure	
Urgency	Number
Elective	10
Scheduled	11
Emergency	98
Emergency (catheter complication)	1
Not answered	1
Total	121

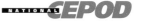

Coexisting medical conditions

Key Point

- *A high proportion of patients had coexisting medical conditions.*

Table 10: Coexisting medical conditions *(121 cases; answers may be multiple)*	
Coexisting condition	**Number**
None	22
A history of raised blood pressure requiring treatment	46
Diabetes	24
Chronic obstructive pulmonary disease/emphysema/asthma: requiring bronchodilator or steroid medication	21
Previous cerebrovascular event	17
Occlusive peripheral vascular disease	12
Renal impairment (creatinine > 200 micromol/l)	11
Active GI problem e.g. peptic ulceration, cholecystitis, diverticulitis	6
Abdominal aortic aneurysm	1
Past history of deep vein thrombosis or pulmonary embolism	1
Dysrhythmia:　　Atrial flutter/fibrillation	9
Ventricular tachycardia	8
Medication for previous ventricular tachycardia	5
Complete heart block	4

There were a large number of coexisting medical problems and in only 22 patients were there no other medical problems apart from the coronary artery disease.

Category of myocardial ischaemia

Key Point

- *Eighty percent of patients were admitted with acute coronary syndromes (unstable angina or acute myocardial infarction).*

Table 11 details the category of myocardial ischaemia. None of those treated was asymptomatic, nor did any patient have acute coronary occlusion following a PTCA. It is interesting to note that 75 procedures (62%) were performed for patients with acute MI and 40 of these were described as being in shock. In a further 22 there was continuing unstable angina and in only 15 did the patient have stable angina. Thus, 97 (80%) patients were admitted with continuing unstable angina or acute MI (acute coronary syndromes); conditions which are recognised as being associated with a significantly increased risk when angioplasty is performed.

Table 11: Category of myocardial ischaemia	
Category	Number
Stable angina	15
Stabilised unstable angina	6
Continuing unstable angina	22
Acute MI without shock	35
Acute MI with shock	40
Not answered	3
Total	121

In the years 1992-1996 approximately 2% of PTCA procedures were for acute MI[4]; by 1997 this had risen to 5%[11] and the number performed acutely continues to rise, supported by a number of studies[13,14].

Extent of coronary artery disease

Key Point

- *The majority of patients had disease in more than one coronary artery.*

Table 12 shows the extent of the coronary artery disease; the majority of patients had disease in more than one coronary artery. Fourteen of the patients had disease in the left main stem (LMS) artery. Until a few years ago angioplasty would not have been attempted in such patients, and especially not to the LMS itself, since it supplies most of the arterial blood supply to the left ventricle and occlusion would almost inevitably result in a fatal infarction. However, in the emergency situation, especially following an acute myocardial infarction, patients with LMS stenosis may undergo PTCA to other lesions or occasionally to the LMS itself.

It is important to point out that the PTCA is not performed on every area of narrowing, but to those that are thought to be responsible for the main problem facing the patient (i.e. the 'culprit lesions'). The fact that there may be LMS disease does not necessarily mean that the patient needs LMS angioplasty. The greater the extent and severity of the coronary disease, the higher the risk of angioplasty; the patients who died were predominantly in the high risk category.

Table 12: Extent of coronary artery disease (121 cases; answers may be multiple)	
Extent of coronary artery disease	Number
Left main stem	14
1 vessel	21
2 vessel	39
3 vessel	55
Other	1
Not answered	1

Left ventricular dysfunction

Key Point

• *A high proportion of patients had moderate or severe left ventricular dysfunction.*

Table 13: Left ventricular dysfunction (prior to procedure)	
Left ventricular dysfunction	Number
None	15
Mild	21
Moderate	18
Severe	42
Not known	6
Not answered	19
Total	121

Table 13 gives details of left ventricular dysfunction prior to the procedure. Of the 96 patients in whom the left ventricular (LV) function was known, almost two thirds (63%) had moderate or severe dysfunction. As LV function is an independent predictor of survival, these patients were at much higher risk than normal before undergoing their PTCA.

Twenty-nine patients had the ejection fraction measured. This is an objective angiographic assessment of LV function, with a normal value of greater than 65%. While this is a routine measurement in patients having elective procedures many cardiologists consider that it is not appropriate in the emergency situation, although others believe it is helpful in subsequent management of the patient. Figure 5 displays the results and shows that where an objective angiographic assessment of LV function was made before the PTCA procedure, the majority of patients had moderate or severe LV impairment.

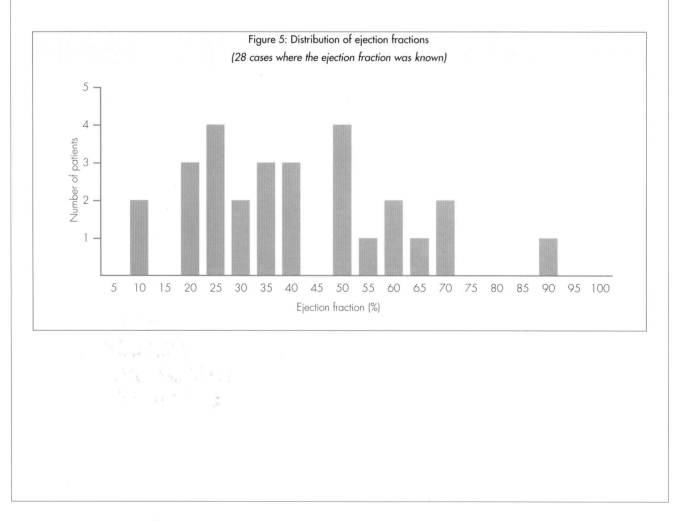

Figure 5: Distribution of ejection fractions
(28 cases where the ejection fraction was known)

Anticipated risk of death

Key Points

- *There was a poor correlation between the assessed risk of death and the stated presence of cardiogenic shock.*
- *There is a need for better understanding of the definition of cardiogenic shock, in order to be able to give an accurate prognosis.*

Those performing the angioplasty were asked to assess the anticipated risk of death for that patient if the PTCA was undertaken (Table 14). There was a difference of opinion between the advisors' assessment of the anticipated risk and the answers given. This may have been due to a possible misunderstanding of the question. It was meant to enquire of the overall risk of the patient dying, but may have been interpreted as the risk of the angioplasty causing the death of the patient. Certainly there was poor correlation between the estimated risk and the presence of cardiogenic shock, a condition with a universally poor outcome (approximately 80% mortality). It may be that there is a poor understanding of the definition of cardiogenic shock. Cardiogenic shock has been variously defined as *"a state of inadequate tissue perfusion due to cardiac dysfunction, most commonly caused by acute myocardial infarction"*[15], or more specifically on the basis of the patient's haemodynamic profile, which may be considered in terms of LV filling pressure, systolic blood pressure or elevated right ventricular filling pressure[16], or cardiac index or pulmonary capillary wedge pressure[17]. However, patients undergoing emergency PTCA are not likely to have time for intensive investigation. There is, therefore, a need for a clear and universally accepted clinical definition, so that accurate risk assessment can be made in order to obtain reliable informed consent.

Since 1987 there has been a formal risk assessment for patients undergoing cardiac surgery for adult acquired heart disease[18]. There is a need to develop a similar risk assessment for PTCA in order to obtain reliable informed consent and to assess comparative results of different units or of various treatments.

Table 14: Anticipated risk of death	
Risk of death	Number
<1%	10
1-5%	23
6-10%	16
11-50%	36
>50%	36
Total	121

Previous coronary artery bypass grafts (CABG)

Nine of the 121 patients had previously undergone CABG (7%). The reason for this low percentage is unknown; however, a relatively small number of angioplasty procedures are performed on grafts in patients who have previously undergone CABG. In 1996 the mean number of angioplasty procedures per intervention centre was 380, whereas only 49 procedures on grafts were performed on average per centre[4].

Restenosis lesions

In only three of the 121 patients was the PTCA performed for a stenosis that had previously been treated by angioplasty and in whom a restenosis had developed.

PROCEDURAL DETAILS

This section reviews the proposed and actual coronary interventions, together with therapeutic manoeuvres prior to the procedure. It also considers the experience and availability of the operator and person with overall responsibility, the type of anaesthesia, cardiac arrest and resuscitation, monitoring, sedation, oxygen therapy and pulse oximetry. The method of anticoagulation and whether monitored with activated clotting time (ACT) is followed by a review of complications and referral for coronary artery bypass grafting (CABG).

Coronary vessel treated

Key Point

- *PTCA was most frequently performed on the left anterior descending (LAD) artery, followed by the right coronary artery (RCA).*

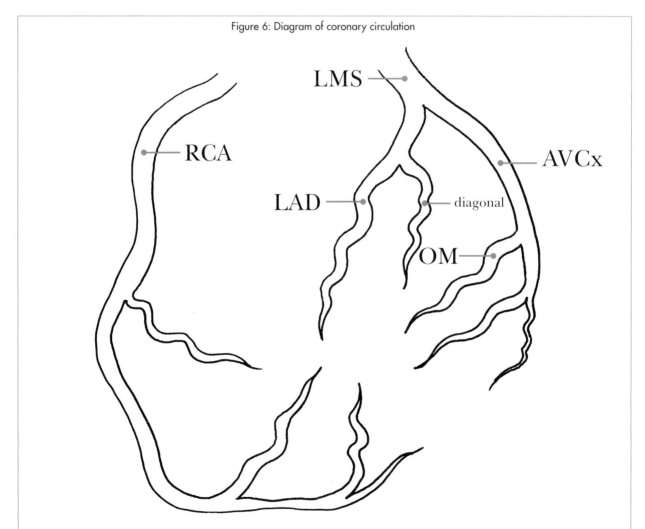

Figure 6: Diagram of coronary circulation

The coronary arteries as if viewed from the apex of the heart. The perimeter of the diagram is the atrioventricular groove.

The two coronaries arising from the aorta are the right (RCA) and the left main stem (LMS) coronary arteries. The left divides within 1-2 cm into the left anterior descending (LAD) and the atrioventricular circumflex (AVCx) arteries. Branches of the LAD supplying the anterolateral part of the left ventricle are called diagonal branches of the LAD. The lateral aspect of the left ventricle is supplied by obtuse marginal (OM) branches of the circumflex system.

Table 15 summarises which coronary arteries were proposed for PTCA, compared with those actually attempted. The vast majority of patients did have dilatation of the vessel proposed prior to the procedure. In a few cases further lesions, in other coronary arteries, were treated for reasons that became apparent during the procedure.

The LAD coronary artery was the most commonly attempted in this group of patients, reflecting the recognised importance of this vessel which supplies the majority of the left ventricle.

Table 15: Proposed and actual coronary artery attempted (121 cases; answers may be multiple)		
Coronary artery	Proposed	Attempted
RCA	38	39
LMS	7	7
AVCx	14	12
OM	10	10
LAD	65	66
Diagonal	5	8
SV graft	6	6
LIMA graft	1	1

Elective stenting

Key Point

* *Intracoronary stents were inserted in approximately 50% of cases.*

The use of an intracoronary stent was planned before the procedure in 58/121 (48%) patients. This percentage is in keeping with data from the BCIS audit where 60% of procedures in 1997 involved the use of a stent[11]. Trials in recent years have shown a lower restenosis rate after stenting compared with angioplasty alone[2, 3]. The National Institute for Clinical Excellence (NICE) has recently reported on the use of intracoronary stents, favouring their use in the majority of angioplasty procedures[19,20].

Therapeutic manoeuvres prior to the procedure

Key Point

* *Intra-aortic balloon pumps would appear to be underused considering the fairly high proportion of patients reported to be in cardiogenic shock.*

Table 16: Therapeutic manoeuvres undertaken before the procedure (121 cases; answers may be multiple)	
Therapeutic manoeuvre	Number
None of note	24
IV nitrates	46
IV heparin	56
IV inotropes	18
Thrombolytic agent (within last 24 hours)	34
IIb/IIIa receptor antagonists	11
Intra-aortic balloon pump (IABP)	24
Mechanical ventilation	10
Antiarrhythmics for previous ventricular tachycardia/ ventricular fibrillation	10
Temporary pacing	16
Other	14

Details of the therapeutic manoeuvres undertaken before the procedure to try and improve the patient's condition are shown in Table 16.

Of note is the fact that only 24/121 (20%) had an intra-aortic balloon pump (IABP) used prior to the procedure. The advisors found this surprising in view of the high number of patients (40) considered to be in cardiogenic shock (Table 11, page 11).

See also page 24 on the use of IABPs following the procedure.

Experience and availability of the operator

Key Points

- *There was very high consultant involvement in these PTCA procedures.*
- *Operators were fully trained and considered to be suitably experienced to perform the procedure in almost all cases.*

Grade of the operator

Table 17 gives details of the first and second operator. A high proportion of the procedures were performed by consultant cardiologists. Almost all of the remainder were undertaken by senior registrars, who by virtue of their seniority, would have been experienced independent operators.

Other commitments

Cardiologists would not normally have other commitments when scheduled to perform coronary interventions. They may, of course, occasionally be called to help in an emergency when they do have other fixed sessions. In practice it seemed to be rare that this was the case (7/121; 6%); however, work plans and rotas for interventionists should be designed to keep this to a minimum.

Table 17: Grade of operator		
Grade	First operator	Second operator
Consultant cardiologist	96	18
Senior registrar cardiology	21	28
Senior registrar radiology	0	2
Specialist registrar	3	48
Other	1	9
Not answered/None	0	16
Total	121	121

Clinical and procedural responsibility

Table 18: Clinical and procedural responsibility	
Consultant involvement	Number
A consultant interventionist was present throughout and performed the procedure	100
A consultant interventionist was present throughout but performed only a small part, or no part, of the procedure	12
A consultant interventionist was immediately available in the hospital for advice but undertook little or no direct part in the procedure	7
A consultant interventionist was immediately available outside the hospital for advice	2
Total	121

Details of the clinical and procedural responsibility are given in Table 18. There were nine cases in which a consultant was not immediately available in the catheter laboratory. The BCIS guidelines[21] state that specialist registrars should perform 200 PTCAs in their final two years of training, 125 of which should be as first operator, before they can be considered for accreditation. They also state that an independent solo operator should perform a minimum of 75 interventions a year to maintain a satisfactory level of skill, though this figure was set at 60/year during the period of this survey.

Of these nine registrars, all had been performing between 100 and 250 cases per year for between two and five years, so that they all fulfilled these criteria.

There were three cases where the advisors raised concerns:

CASE 9 • *A 70-year-old patient admitted as an emergency with an MI had the procedure performed by an experienced SpR who had been a solo operator for three years and had performed 250 interventions in the previous year. He was assisted by a less experienced registrar. An obtuse marginal coronary artery ruptured and the patient died of cardiac tamponade. Although this registrar was very experienced, the fact that there was no consultant present at any stage was considered to be less than ideal in what was a very difficult situation.*

CASE 10 • *A 55-year-old patient was transferred from a DGH with an MI and cardiogenic shock. PTCA of the LAD was attempted by an SpR supervised by a consultant, but failed. The patient became progressively more hypotensive and died during the procedure. Although the outcome would almost certainly have been the same, this was not thought to be an appropriate case for teaching purposes.*

CASE 11 • *51-year-old patient with crippling stable angina whose general condition was so poor that she needed domiciliary oxygen and a Zimmer frame. The procedure on this poor risk patient was started by a cardiology registrar, although the consultant did come to help when difficulties developed. This was not considered to be an ideal patient to delegate to a trainee.*

Despite these criticisms, overall the advisors were impressed with the high level of consultant involvement in these difficult cases.

Experience of the operator

Key Point

• *The majority of cardiologists (95%) are complying with the BCIS recommendations on the number of procedures which should be performed each year.*

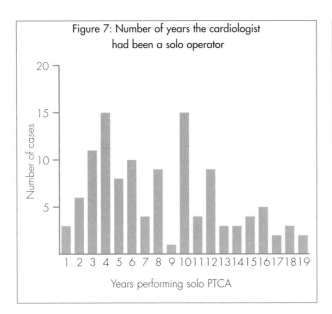

Figure 7: Number of years the cardiologist had been a solo operator

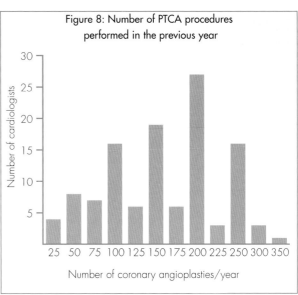

Figure 8: Number of PTCA procedures performed in the previous year

Figures 7 and 8 show that in three cases the operator had a year or less of solo experience, and in 12 the number of procedures performed in the previous year was less than 75, the number currently recommended by BCIS as the minimum to be performed each year by an independent solo operator. At the time the information for this report was collected the recommended minimum was 60, and in six cases the operator had performed less than 60 PTCA procedures in the previous year. The question was answered in 116 cases; thus, 110/116 (95%) had performed 60 or more cases in the previous year.

One case is worthy of mention:

CASE 12 • *A 52-year-old patient admitted as an emergency with an MI and cardiogenic shock had a PTCA of the LAD. Clot propagated back to the left main stem artery with fatal outcome. The operator had performed only 25 procedures in the previous year.*

The view of the advisors was that this person did not have enough experience to take on such a sick patient, and a system should be established such that there is always a sufficiently experienced cardiologist available.

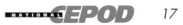

Anaesthesia

Key Point

- *There should be a designated person to check that all necessary equipment is present and functional.*

One hundred and nine procedures (90%) were performed under local anaesthetic; ten were performed under general anaesthesia. An anaesthetist was also present for a further 11 cases performed under local anaesthetic. It was thought that this would usually be because the patient had respiratory problems or had suffered a cardiac arrest. There was cause for concern in one case:

CASE 13 • *A 72-year-old patient admitted as an emergency with an acute MI and cardiogenic shock required ventilation. There was said to be "inadequate airway and anaesthetic equipment". Oxygen had been given but a pulse oximeter was not used to monitor the adequacy of oxygenation.*

Administering anaesthesia in an angiography suite is not straightforward. It is essential that the facilities for managing the airway and all other anaesthetic equipment are checked regularly to ensure that they are present and working. It is preferable for this to be done by an operating department practitioner from the main operating theatre suite. A trained anaesthetic assistant is needed to help the anaesthetist; this is particularly important in the catheter laboratory, being a more difficult environment than the operating theatre and distant from other immediate anaesthetic assistance.

Resuscitation

Key Point

- *Ninety-four percent of catheter laboratory staff receive regular resuscitation training; while recognising that this is commendably high, the figure should be 100%.*

Regular resuscitation training was reported in 114/121 questionnaires received. In only three was it stated that this did not occur, while in a further four it was not known or not answered. It is essential that catheter laboratory staff have regular resuscitation training. Indeed this is already occurring in almost all departments (94%).

Cardiac arrest occurred during the final procedure in 26/121 reported cases. In all 26, the person filling in the questionnaire considered that resuscitation was performed to a satisfactory standard. In three cases the patient was resuscitated, stabilised and then transferred for CABG.

Monitoring, sedation and oxygen therapy

Key Points

- *Monitoring with pulse oximetry should be available for all cases and performed whenever sedation or opiates are used or oxygen therapy is required.*
- *An appropriately trained nurse or technician should be responsible for monitoring, and not the cardiologist performing the procedure*

Premedication was given to 33/121 patients. Thirty-nine patients had sedation given during the procedure, 17 of whom had also had a premedication. Twenty-four of those having sedation also received opiates, as did a further 14 non-sedated patients. Ninety-one patients (75%) were given oxygen therapy.

Pulse oximetry

Pulse oximetry was monitored in 82 patients (68%). All patients routinely have the ECG and blood pressure monitored closely. A significant proportion of patients had a premedication (27%), sedation (32%) and/or opiates. It is particularly important in these patients that pulse oximetry is monitored, and oxygen therapy should be available for all patients[22]. It can be argued that pulse oximetry is not needed if the patient is not having oxygen or sedation and is stable, but it is helpful if the patient deteriorates and, of course, one does not know when this may happen. Table 21 (page 21) lists the complications of the final PTCA procedures. It is interesting to note that of the 16 patients who were recorded as having hypoxaemia, 13 of them were monitored with pulse oximetry. In one it was not known whether or not this was the case, but in two pulse oximetry was definitely not monitored. Similarly, of the 24 patients who needed ventilation, 21 had pulse oximetry performed, in one it was not known and in two it was not performed.

Although the BCIS guidelines[21] recommend that pulse oximetry should always be available, they fall short of saying it should always be used. The NCEPOD cardiology advisors were not unanimous on this point, although the anaesthetic advisors were. It is a very simple thing to do, is unobtrusive and can be set with its own alarm, and seems a sensible routine precaution.

Table 19 details who was responsible for monitoring pulse oximetry. It is inappropriate for monitoring to be the responsibility of the cardiologist performing the procedure, which may frequently be technically demanding. Most catheter laboratories have cardiac technicians and nurses present during PTCA, and one of these, suitably trained, should be identified as having responsibility for monitoring pulse oximetry, as indeed was the case in the majority (80%).

Table 19: Responsibility for monitoring pulse oximetry	
Person responsible	Number
Operator	8
Nurse	54
Technician	12
Radiographer	2
Other	5
Not answered	1
Total	82

Anticoagulants

Key Point

- *There appears to be an under-use of glycoprotein IIb/IIIa receptor blockers. These should be used more widely in patients undergoing high risk PTCA. Heparin doses should be adjusted accordingly, and monitored using activated clotting time (ACT) or equivalent, in order to minimise the risk of bleeding.*

Anticoagulant	Before	During	After
Heparin	83	79	31
Aspirin	102	17	29
Thrombolytic treatment	35	1	0
Oral IIb/IIIa antagonist	1	6	2
Intravenous IIb/IIIa antagonist	6	32	20
Ticlopidine	9	5	29
Clopidogrel	8	3	18
Oral anticoagulant	1	0	0
Other	1	2	0
Not answered	4	26	57

Table 20: Anticoagulant treatment given before, during or after the procedure
(121 cases; answers may be multiple)

Table 20 gives details of anticoagulant treatment given before, during or after the procedure. A relatively small number of patients were given the intravenous IIb/IIIa antagonist abciximab (ReoPro). This drug has been shown to improve the results both for PTCA and for stent application[7,8]. However, the data for this study were collected from 1 September 1998 to 31 August 1999, when its use was less common; usage of the drug is increasing.

Activated clotting time

The advisors considered it important to measure the activated clotting time (ACT) or equivalent to monitor the amount of heparin used. This was carried out in 65/121 cases (54%); in 47 it was not and in a further nine it was not known. Most cardiologists now use weight-adjusted heparin in case they wish to use abciximab. The individual response of patients is variable, with some patients getting high levels of ACT with relatively low doses of heparin. Some clinicians use abciximab before they start the case, while others give it when they think it is needed during the case. Heparin doses should be adjusted accordingly, and monitored with ACT or equivalent, in order to minimise the risk of bleeding. An example is given:

CASE 14 • *A 65-year-old patient with an acute MI and associated cardiogenic shock had an attempted angioplasty of the RCA. He had been given heparin and at the end of the procedure was given abciximab, but without first measuring the ACT. He almost certainly did have coagulation problems because he developed a large haematoma in the neck at the site of an intravenous line and apparently had significant blood loss.*

Success of the procedure

Forty-seven percent (57/121) of the cases were apparently not completed satisfactorily and/or had a complication; this seems a very high proportion. However, the advisors had the impression that where patients had deteriorated, and sometimes died in the catheter laboratory, as a consequence of their severe condition, many of these cases were being reported as unsatisfactory and/or complicated. They did not consider that the angioplasty procedure itself had caused the complication or unsatisfactory outcome. Of course, no matter how well the procedure had gone from a technical point of view, if the patient died it could not be recorded as anything other than an 'unsatisfactory outcome'.

A more detailed analysis was performed to try and find any common factors that were associated with the operator's interpretation of a complication or unsatisfactory procedure but nothing obvious came to light.

Complications

Key Point

• *The high proportion of complications reflects the large number of patients admitted with acute myocardial infarction and cardiogenic shock.*

Table 21: Complications of the final PTCA procedure (121 cases; answers may be multiple)	
Complication	Number
Coronary (e.g. coronary thrombosis, dissection, coronary rupture, acute occlusion, loss of side branch)	43
Hypotension (requiring inotropes and/or IABP)	43
Cardiac arrest	28
Bradycardia (requiring pacing)	28
Need for ventilation	24
Hypoxaemia	16
Tachyarrhythmias	11
Technical (relating to equipment e.g. lost stent/wire fragment)	5
Other	11
Not answered	23
None	6
Total	121

Details of the various complications that developed during the final procedure are shown in Table 21.

The incidence of coronary complications seems quite high (36%), but bearing in mind that in many of these the artery was occluded before the procedure began, as would commonly be the case in patients with acute infarction, and over 80% of them were done as an emergency, this accounts for the results. Most of the complications reported were probably events that were observed during the procedure, but which were part of the syndrome being treated, rather than actual complications. It should be remembered that the emergency group, if they have conventional medical treatment without attempts at revascularisation, have a high mortality, particularly those who have cardiogenic shock where the mortality is about 80%[15].

Cardiac enzymes

Table 22: Measurement of cardiac enzymes		
	Cardiac enzymes measured following PTCA in this case	Cardiac enzymes measured routinely following PTCA procedures
Yes	49	58
No	64	60
Not answered	8	3
Total	121	121

Table 22 indicates whether cardiac enzymes were measured in the particular case being reported, and also whether it was the cardiologist's practice to measure them routinely after all PTCA procedures. Many of these cases were being undertaken in the context of acute myocardial infarction where cardiac enzymes would be measured on a daily basis, but not necessarily following the angioplasty procedure. However, centres are encouraged to measure cardiac enzymes following PTCA as a routine, being part of the data set required by the Central Cardiac Audit Database project, a national data collection exercise supported by the Department of Health, the British Cardiac Society, BCIS, the Society of Cardiothoracic Surgeons and the Association of Cardiothoracic Anaesthetists.

Referral for cardiac surgery

Key Point

- *Very few patients underwent emergency or urgent CABG following PTCA.*

Availability of emergency cardiac surgery

All centres performing coronary angioplasty procedures had access to emergency cardiac surgery; this complies with national guidelines[21]. In 113/121 (93%) cases this was on the same site, in six (5%) it was at a different hospital and in two the question was not answered.

While it may be simpler if interventional cardiology and cardiac surgery are on the same site, the guidelines[21] state that, providing the patient can be transferred to the cardiac surgical unit, and be on cardiopulmonary bypass, within ninety minutes of the request from the catheter laboratory, this is considered to be acceptable, whether it is in the same hospital or involving an ambulance transfer.

Discussion with a specific cardiac surgeon before undertaking the procedure

In only 27/121 (22%) cases was there a discussion with a specific cardiac surgeon prior to embarking on the PTCA procedure. The majority of these patients had their angioplasty procedure as an emergency, mainly for acute myocardial infarction. In these circumstances it is generally accepted that urgent coronary bypass surgery is rarely an alternative treatment, and hence the majority of patients were not discussed with a surgeon. Indeed, although close collaboration between cardiologists and cardiac surgeons is expected[21], it is not a requirement that all cases are discussed.

Referral for coronary artery bypass grafts (CABG)

Ten patients were referred for CABG. Of these, four were transferred as an emergency from the catheter laboratory, two were transferred later but within 24 hours, and a further two had surgery after more than 24 hours but during the same admission. The remaining two did not ultimately have surgery performed and none was readmitted for surgery at a later date. The advisors had anticipated that the study might demonstrate a significant proportion of those patients who died having been referred for emergency CABG if the PTCA procedure had

failed. The fact that there were only four reflects the high percentage who had the angioplasty performed for acute MI, where emergency CABG is rarely helpful in patient management.

There was an inappropriate delay in CABG being undertaken in one case:

CASE 15 • *A 61-year-old patient with continuing unstable angina had a failed RCA angioplasty which caused a dissection of this vessel and of the aorta. There was a delay of over three hours because both cardiac theatres were in use with elective work. The patient was kept alive by the use of an IABP. During this time she had four cardiac arrests, from which she was successfully resuscitated, but which would have lessened her chances of survival.*

Another case of interest was:

CASE 13 • *A 72-year-old patient had already been assessed and turned down for cardiac surgery and was subsequently admitted as an emergency with acute MI and cardiogenic shock. The cardiologist felt that it was right to try an angioplasty as his only hope of survival, but this proved to be technically impossible. The surgeon actually obtained consent from the patient and when he deteriorated it was the surgeon who intubated the trachea and commented on the lack of anaesthetic facilities. The patient survived the operation, but died six days later (see also page 18).*

It is not uncommon for patients turned down for cardiac surgery to be taken on by a cardiologist for coronary intervention. The question arises as to whether it is really appropriate to go back to considering cardiac surgery if the PTCA fails?

The small number of surgical and anaesthetic questionnaires returned in relation to those patients having CABG operations were studied by the advisors, but yielded no significant additional information.

POSTPROCEDURAL CARE

Key Point

- *A designated recovery area was available in 81% of cases.*

Destination following catheter laboratory

Table 23 summarises where the patients went after leaving the catheter laboratory. The majority were cared for in some form of higher dependency area following their PTCA.

Designated and equipped recovery area

A designated and fully equipped recovery area was available in 98/121 (81%) cases. It was the advisors' view that a recovery area should be available for all patients.

Length of stay

Table 24 summarises the average number of days patients spent on respective wards. This confirms an earlier comment (page 4), indicating that those patients dying following PTCA usually do so within a few days of the procedure.

Table 23: Destination of the patient on leaving the catheter laboratory	
Destination	Number
Cardiac theatre for emergency CABG	4
CCU	58
HDU	6
ICU	19
Recovery room	2
Cardiac ward	11
General ward	1
Died in the catheter laboratory	17
Other	2
Not answered	1
Total	121

Table 24: Number of days on respective wards			
(98 patients who did not die in the catheter laboratory or undergo CABG within 24 hours; answers may be multiple)			
Ward	Total number of days	Number of patients	Mean number of days/patient
CCU	153	57	2.7
ICU	77	18	4.3
HDU	17	8	2.1
Cardiac ward	116	20	5.8
General ward	3	3	1
Not answered	-	10	-

Drugs used following PTCA

Table 25 gives details of intravenous drugs used following the PTCA. These are all standard drugs used for patients following angioplasty and/or those with an acute MI. The increasing use of IIb/IIIa antagonists (abciximab) has already been commented upon (page 20).

Table 25: Intravenous drugs used following PTCA	
(98 patients who did not die in the catheter laboratory or undergo CABG within 24 hours; answers may be multiple)	
Drug	Number
Heparin	44
Nitrates	30
IIb/IIIa antagonists	32
Inotropes	40
Renal dopamine	23
Other	5
Not answered	21
None	5

Other supportive measures following PTCA

Key Points

- *Intra-aortic balloon pumps would appear to be under-used considering the fairly high proportion of patients reported to be in cardiogenic shock.*

- *Staff caring for patients after PTCA procedures should be familiar with the use of the intra-aortic balloon pump (IABP); these should be functional, and reserve machines should be available.*

Table 26: Other supportive measures following PTCA
(98 patients who did not die in the catheter laboratory or undergo CABG within 24 hours; answers may be multiple)

Supportive measure	Number
IABP	31
Ventilation	17
Pacing	10
CVVH/dialysis	3
Intracoronary infusion	1
Not answered	54
None	5

Although an intra-aortic balloon pump (IABP) was used in 31 (32%) cases (Table 26) the view of the advisors was that it should perhaps have been used more often (see also page 15). There were three cases where patients were in cardiogenic shock and no IABP was used. In each instance the advisors thought that it might well have helped:

CASE 16 • *A 65-year-old patient with cardiogenic shock due to an acute MI had to be nursed on the ICU because there was no CCU bed available. The staff were not familiar with the IABP and so did not use one even though it might have helped. There appeared to be an excessive use of adrenaline and a pulmonary artery catheter should have been considered.*

CASE 17 • *A 67-year-old patient with an acute MI and cardiogenic shock. An IABP machine failed at time of insertion and no other balloon pump was available.*

CASE 18 • *A 76-year-old patient with an acute MI and cardiogenic shock had persistent hypotension despite all treatment. A balloon pump was not used, but might have helped.*

Hindrances and complications in postprocedural management

Hindrances

There were four patients of the 98 (4%), in whom there were factors which hindered the clinical management following the procedure. In three it was the lack or failure of a balloon pump (cases 16, 17 and 18).

CASE 19 • *A 67-year-old patient had a PTCA of the LAD and diagonal artery. She had rheumatoid arthritis and developed a false aneurysm at the femoral artery puncture site; she also had suspected atlanto-axial subluxation which made endotracheal intubation more difficult when she suffered a cardiac arrest.*

Complications

Table 27: Clinical complications
(66 cases; answers may be multiple)

Complication	Number
Cardiac arrest	34
Renal failure	11
Stroke	7
Electrolyte derangement	6
Respiratory failure	5
Acute abdomen	2
Sepsis	2
Haemorrhage from arterial access site	1
Aneurysm of access site	1
Loss of arterial supply to limb	1
Requirement for vascular surgery	1
Hepatic failure	1
Urinary tract infection	1
Other	14
Not answered	1

Of the 115 patients who did not go on to have a CABG within the first 24 hours, 66 of them (57%) had clinical complications of one sort or another, while only 26 had no complications (in the remaining 23 cases the question was not answered). Table 27 summarises these complications.

The question asked whether there were any haematological disorders; it is interesting to note that none was recorded, despite the fact that a high proportion of the patients had had streptokinase, heparin and antiplatelet drugs. However, one patient had haemorrhage from the arterial access site and, of the 14 described as 'other', at least five almost certainly had coagulation problems. It is also interesting to note that there were no cases of DVT or pulmonary embolism, probably reflecting the frequent use of anticoagulants or antiplatelet drugs.

The 14 complications listed as 'other' were:

- Epistaxis and haemoptysis; abciximab infusion had to be stopped after eight hours
- Lung haemorrhage
- Gastrointestinal bleeding
- Gastrointestinal bleed & extension of cerebral infarct
- Unexplained decrease in haemoglobin to 6 g/dl
- Hypotension
- Pneumothorax and pulmonary oedema
- Above knee amputation for lower limb ischaemia
- Acute stent occlusion two hours after the procedure
- Chest infection
- Severe left ventricular failure
- Cardiac tamponade due to rupture of infarcted heart muscle
- Pneumonia
- Cardiogenic shock

Cardiopulmonary resuscitation

Key Point

- *The decision whether or not cardiopulmonary resuscitation (CPR) should be performed was made in a responsible way by experienced cardiologists.*

Cardiopulmonary resuscitation (CPR) was attempted in 62/121 (51%) patients; in 47 it was not attempted, while in a further 12 the answer was not known or not given. In 12 of these 47 for whom CPR was not attempted, it was recorded that the decision was made prior to the procedure.

Further analysis of these 12 cases revealed that ten of the patients were already in cardiogenic shock. The other two developed cardiogenic shock slightly later and, in fact, after the procedure had been performed. It was thought likely in these cases that the decision not to resuscitate was actually made before the cardiac arrest, if not actually prior to the initial procedure. However, in all cases the patients were in cardiogenic shock. While every effort should be made to try and improve their condition, if deterioration continues until cardiac arrest occurs, under these circumstances there is no chance of successful resuscitation. It was, therefore, a reasonable decision.

In two of the twelve cases it was not known who made the decision not to resuscitate, in a further two it was an experienced SpR 4 and in the remaining eight the decision was made by a consultant cardiologist.

DEATH

Place of death

Table 28: Place of death	
Place	Number
Catheter laboratory	17
Theatre suite	4
ICU	27
HDU	6
CCU	45
Cardiac ward	10
General ward	2
Other hospital	1
Out of hospital	6
Other	1
Not answered	2
Total	121

Postmortem examinations

Key Points

- *Clinicians should be informed of the date and time that postmortem examinations are being performed and should make every effort to attend.*

- *A copy of the postmortem report should always be sent to the appropriate clinician.*

- *In almost one in four of the postmortem examinations performed the pathological findings differed from the clinical impression, emphasising why it is important that they be performed.*

In 79/121 (65%) cases the death was reported to the coroner, but a coroner's postmortem examination was only performed in 31 cases. Of the 90 cases in whom a coroner's postmortem was not performed, a hospital postmortem was only carried out in seven (8%).

In 28/38 cases a consultant pathologist performed the postmortem examination; in three cases it was a junior pathologist and in a further seven it was not answered or not known. In 19 cases the postmortem was carried out by a general pathologist, in three by a cardiac pathologist, in one by a Home Office pathologist and in a further 15 it was not known or not answered.

Of the 38 postmortem examinations that were performed, the cardiologist was only informed of the date and time in 14 cases (37%). Table 29 shows the clinicians who attended the postmortem examination.

It is commendable that in 9/14 cases where they were aware of the postmortem examination, at least one member of the clinical team attended; it is disappointing that they were not informed of the time and date in so many instances.

Table 29: Members of the team attending the postmortem examination (14 cases where the clinical team was informed; in one case two clinicians attended the postmortem)	
Grade	Number
Consultant	3
SpR	5
SHO	1
Other	1
Not known	1
None	4

Table 30: Receipt of copy of the postmortem report by the clinical team	
Report received	Number
Yes	24
No	6
Informal report or verbal message only	7
Not answered	1
Total	38

It is disappointing that in six cases (16%) the clinicians did not receive a copy of the postmortem report at all, and in a further seven (18%) only a verbal report was obtained.

Twenty-three of the 38 postmortem examinations confirmed the cardiology team's clinical impression; in eight the question was not answered, but in seven the postmortem did not confirm the clinical team's impression. Two patients who were thought clinically to have had a pulmonary embolism, were shown at postmortem to have died from coronary occlusion. One patient had a rupture of the obtuse marginal coronary artery which caused cardiac tamponade; this was not recognised at the time, and was an unexpected finding at postmortem. A second patient also had cardiac tamponade, due to rupture of necrotic and infarcted heart muscle. One patient was thought to have dissected and occluded the LAD; at postmortem the vessel was completely clear, although the patient did die of ischaemic heart disease despite this. Conversely there was a further patient in whom it was thought that a left main stem angioplasty had been successful, but at postmortem there was a dissection and the vessel had occluded. One further patient was said to have postmortem findings at variance with the clinical team's impression, but no further details were given.

This underlines the reasons why postmortem examinations are of educational benefit.

AUDIT MEETINGS AND AVAILABILITY OF CASE NOTES

Key Points

- *In 92% of cases the interventional centres held regular audit meetings; those not holding such meetings should do so.*
- *With the introduction of clinical governance, case notes should always be readily available.*

Regular audit meetings were held in 111/121 (92%) cases, although only 93 (77%) of the deaths reported in this study were actually considered at a local audit meeting.

While 92% is commendably high, nevertheless those centres that are not holding regular audit meetings should do so and all deaths following PTCA procedures should be considered at such meetings.

There was a problem obtaining case notes, with a delay of more than a week, in 33 cases (27%). In 14 cases (12%) the hospital notes were incomplete. It is to be hoped that with the advent of clinical governance this unsatisfactory situation will improve.

REFERENCES

1. Chauhan A, Vu E, Ricci DR, Buller CE, Moscovich MD, Monkman S, Penn IM. *Early and intermediate term clinical outcome after multiple coronary stenting.* Heart 1998; **79**(1):29-33.

2. Serruys PW, de Jaegere P, Kiemeneij F, Macaya C, Rutsch W, Heyndrickx G, Emanuelsson H, Marco J, Legrand V, Materne P. *A comparison of balloon-expandable-stent implantation with balloon angioplasty in patients with coronary artery disease.* Benestent Study Group. N Eng J Med 1994; **331**(8):489-95.

3. Fischman DL, Leon MB, Baim DS, Schatz RA, Savage MP, Penn I, Detre K, Veltri L, Ricci D, Nobuyoshi M et al. *A randomized comparison of coronary-stent placement and balloon angioplasty in the treatment of coronary artery disease.* Stent Restenosis Study. N Eng J Med 1994; **331**(8):496-501.

4. Gray HH. *Cardiac interventional procedures in the UK 1992 to 1996.* Council of the British Cardiovascular Intervention Society. Heart 2000; **82** Suppl 2:II10-17.

5. Grines CL, Cox DA, Stone GW, Garcia E, Mattos LA, Giambartolomei A, Brodie BR, Madonna O, Eijgelshoven M, Lansky AJ, O'Neill WW, Morice M; for the Stent Primary Angioplasty in Myocardial Infarction Study Group. *Coronary angioplasty with or without stent implantation for acute myocardial infarction.* N Eng J Med 1999; **341**:1949-1956.

6. Topol EJ, Ferguson JJ, Weisman HF, Tcheng JE, Ellis SG, Kleiman NS, Ivanhoe RJ, Wang AL, Miller DP, Anderson KM, Califf RM; for the EPIC Investigator Group. *Long term protection from myocardial ischemic events in a randomized trial of brief integrin B3 blockade with percutaneous coronary intervention.* JAMA 1997; **278**:479-484.

7. The EPISTENT Investigators. *Randomised placebo-controlled and balloon-angioplasty-controlled trial to assess safety of coronary stenting with use of platelet glycoprotein-IIb/IIIa blockade.* Lancet 1998; **352**:87-92.

8. The CAPTURE Investigators. *Randomised placebo-controlled trial of abciximab before and during coronary intervention in refractory unstable angina: the CAPTURE study.* Lancet 1997; **349**:1429-1435.

9. Ohman EM, George BS, White CJ et al, and the Randomized IABP Study Group. *Use of aortic counterpulsion to improve sustained coronary artery patency during acute myocardial infarction: results of a randomized trial.* Circulation 1994; **90**:793-9.

10. Ishihara M, Sato H, Tateishi H et al. *Intra-aortic balloon pumping as adjunctive therapy to rescue coronary angioplasty after failed thrombolysis in anterior wall acute myocardial infarction.* Am J Cardiol 1995; **76**:73-5.

11. de Belder MA. *Cardiac intervention procedures in the United Kingdom 1997: developments in data collection.* Council of the British Cardiovascular Intervention Society. Heart 2000; **82** Suppl 2:II2-9.

12. Straumann E, Yoon S, Naegeli B, Frielingsdorf J, Gerber A, Schuiki E, Bertel O. *Hospital transfer for primary coronary angioplasty in high risk patients with acute myocardial infarction.* Heart 1999; **82**(4):415-9.

13. Weaver WD, Simes RJ, Betrui A et al. *Comparison of primary coronary angioplasty and intravenous thrombolytic therapy for acute myocardial infarction.* JAMA 1997; **278**:2093-8.

14. Cucherat M, Bonnefoy E, Tremau G. *Primary angioplasty versus intravenous thrombolysis for acute myocardial infarction (Cochrane Review).* In: The Cochrane Library, Issue 1, 2000. Oxford: Update Software.

15. Hollenberg SM, Kavinsky CJ, Parrillo JE. *Cardiogenic shock.* Annals of Internal Medicine 1999; **131**(1):47-59.

16. McGhie AI, Golstein RA. *Pathogenesis and management of acute heart failure and cardiogenic shock: role of inotropic therapy.* Chest 1992; **102**(5 Suppl 2):626S-632S.

17. Wampler RK, Frazier OH, Lansing AM, Smalling RW, Nicklas JM, Phillips SJ, Guyton RA, Golding LA. *Treatment of cardiogenic shock with the Hemopump left ventricular assist device.* Annals of Thoracic Surgery 1991; **52**(3):506-13.

18. Parsonnet V, Dean D, Bernstein AD. *A method of uniform stratification of risk for evaluating the results of surgery in acquired heart disease.* Circulation 1989; **79**:I3-112.

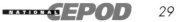

19. Gershlick AH. *Evidence based data to support the use of stents in clinical practice.* Council of BCIS, 1999. www.bcis.org.uk

20. *Guidance on the use of coronary artery stents in the treatment of ischaemic heart disease.* NICE Technology Appraisal Guidance No 4. May 2000. www.nice.org.uk

21. *Coronary angioplasty: guidelines for good practice and training.* Joint Working Group on Coronary Angioplasty of the British Cardiac Society and British Cardiovascular Intervention Society. Heart 2000; **83**(2):224-35.

22. *Guidelines for sedation by non-anaesthetists.* Royal College of Surgeons of England. London, 1993.

Useful web sites

British Cardiac Society	Professional society principally representing UK cardiologists	www.bcs.com
British Cardiovascular Intervention Society (BCIS)	Specialist UK society involved with cardiac intervention procedures	www.bcis.org.uk
British Heart Foundation	UK medical charity supporting cardiovascular research	www.bhf.org.uk
Central Cardiac Audit Database (CCAD)	National cardiac audit database supported by existing UK registries in cardiovascular medicine and surgery	ccad3.biomed.gla.ac.uk/ccad
Commission for Health Improvement (CHI)	Independent statutory body to raise standards throughout NHS in England and Wales	www.doh.gov.uk/chi
Department of Health	Department of Health in England	www.doh.gov.uk
National Institute for Clinical Excellence	Agency setting standards and guidelines for UK medical practice	www.nice.org.uk
Medical Devices Agency	Government agency controlling use of medical devices, including angioplasty equipment	www.medical-devices.gov.uk
Resuscitation Council (UK)	Statements and reports, 1997 resuscitation guidelines	www.resus.org.uk
Royal College of Physicians (London)		www.rcplondon.ac.uk
Scottish Intercollegiate Guidelines Network (SIGN)	National clinical guidelines recommended for use in Scotland. Includes coronary angioplasty	www.show.scot.nhs.uk/sign
Society of Cardiothoracic Surgeons of Great Britain and Ireland	Events, affiliated organisations, training, outcomes, registries and databases	www.scts.org
Journals:		
British Medical Journal		www.bmj.com
Heart (formerly the British Heart Journal)		www.heartjnl.com
Lancet		www.thelancet.com
New England Journal of Medicine		www.nejm.com

APPENDIX A - ABBREVIATIONS

A&E	Accident and Emergency	SVT	Supraventricular tachycardia
ACT	Activated clotting time	VT	Ventricular tachycardia
AVCx	Atrioventricular circumflex (coronary artery)		
BCIS	British Cardiovascular Intervention Society		
CABG	Coronary artery bypass grafts		
CCU	Coronary care unit		
CPR	Cardiopulmonary resuscitation		
CVVH	Continuous venovenous haemofiltration		
DGH	District general hospital		
DVT	Deep vein thrombosis		
ECG	Electrocardiogram		
GI	Gastrointestinal		
HDU	High dependency unit		
IABP	Intra-aortic balloon pump		
ICU	Intensive care unit		
IHD	Ischaemic heart disease		
IV	Intravenous		
LAD	Left anterior descending (coronary artery)		
LIMA	Left internal mammary artery		
LMS	Left main stem (coronary artery)		
LV	Left ventricular		
MI	Myocardial infarction		
OM	Obtuse marginal (coronary artery)		
PTCA	Percutaneous transluminal coronary angioplasty		
RCA	Right coronary artery		
SpR	Specialist registrar		
SV	Saphenous vein		

Appendix B - NCEPOD
Corporate structure

The National Confidential Enquiry into Perioperative Deaths (NCEPOD) is an independent body to which a corporate commitment has been made by the Associations, Colleges and Faculties related to its areas of activity. Each of these bodies nominates members of the Steering Group.

Steering Group
(as at 1 October 2000)

Chairman
Mr John Ll Williams

Members

Mrs M Beck	*(Royal College of Ophthalmologists)*
Dr J F Dyet	*(Royal College of Radiologists)*
Dr H H Gray	*(Royal College of Physicians of London)*
Dr P Kishore	*(Faculty of Public Health Medicine)*
Mr G T Layer	*(Association of Surgeons of Great Britain and Ireland)*
Professor V J Lund	*(Royal College of Surgeons of England)*
Dr J M Millar	*(Royal College of Anaesthetists)*
Dr A J Mortimer	*(Royal College of Anaesthetists)*
Professor J H Shepherd	*(Royal College of Obstetricians and Gynaecologists)*
Dr P J Simpson	*(Royal College of Anaesthetists)*
Mr M F Sullivan	*(Royal College of Surgeons of England)*
Professor P G Toner	*(Royal College of Pathologists)*
Professor T Treasure	*(Royal College of Surgeons of England)*
Dr D J Wilkinson	*(Association of Anaesthetists of Great Britain and Ireland)*
Mr J Ll Williams	*(Faculty of Dental Surgery, Royal College of Surgeons of England)*

Observers

Mr P Milligan	*(Institute of Health Services Management)*
Dr P A Knapman	*(Coroners' Society of England and Wales)*

NCEPOD is a company limited by guarantee, and a registered charity, managed by Trustees.

Trustees

Chairman	Mr J Ll Williams
Treasurer	Dr J N Lunn
	Dr J Lumley
	Dr P J Simpson
	Mr M F Sullivan

Clinical Coordinators

The Steering Group appoint the Principal Clinical Coordinators for a defined tenure. The Principal Clinical Coordinators lead the review of the data relating to the annual sample, advise the Steering Group and write the reports. They may also from time to time appoint Clinical Coordinators, who must be engaged in active academic/clinical practice (in the NHS) during the full term of office.

Principal Clinical Coordinators

Anaesthesia	Dr G S Ingram
Surgery	Mr R W Hoile

Clinical Coordinators

Anaesthesia	Dr A J G Gray
	Dr K M Sherry
Surgery	Mr K G Callum
	Mr I C Martin

Funding

The total annual cost of NCEPOD is approximately £500,000 (1999/2000). We are pleased to acknowledge the support of the following, who contributed to funding the Enquiry in 1999/2000.

National Institute for Clinical Excellence
Welsh Office
Health and Social Services Executive (Northern Ireland)
States of Guernsey Board of Health
States of Jersey
Department of Health and Social Security, Isle of Man Government
Aspen Healthcare
BMI Healthcare
BUPA
Community Hospitals Group
Nuffield Hospitals
PPP/Columbia Healthcare
Benenden Hospital
King Edward VII Hospital, Midhurst
King Edward VII's Hospital for Officers, London
St Martin's Hospitals
The Heart Hospital
The London Clinic

This funding covers the total cost of the Enquiry, including administrative salaries and reimbursements for Clinical Coordinators, office accommodation charges, computer and other equipment as well as travelling and other expenses for the Coordinators, Steering Group and advisory groups.

APPENDIX C - DATA COLLECTION AND REVIEW METHODS

The National Confidential Enquiry into Perioperative Deaths (NCEPOD) reviews clinical practice and aims to identify remediable factors in the practice of anaesthesia, all types of surgery and other invasive procedures. The Enquiry considers the quality of the delivery of care and not specifically causation of death. The commentary in the reports is based on peer review of the data, questionnaires and notes submitted; it is not a research study based on differences against a control population, and does not attempt to produce any kind of comparison between clinicians or hospitals.

The concept of a one-year study reviewing percutaneous transluminal coronary angioplasty (PTCA) represented a unique opportunity for collaboration between NCEPOD and the Royal College of Physicians. The study was also one of the first by NCEPOD to specifically collect denominator data on the total number of procedures performed.

The data collection and review methods are described below.

Scope

All National Health Service hospitals undertaking PTCA in England, Scotland, Wales and Northern Ireland, together with relevant hospitals in the independent sector, were invited to participate in the study.

The period for which data was collected ran from 1 September 1998 to 31 August 1999 and participation was voluntary, being before the introduction of clinical governance and any requirement to take part in this type of Enquiry.

Data collection and review

All relevant hospitals were invited, via a local member of the British Cardiovascular Intervention Society (BCIS), to participate in the study and to nominate a suitable person to take responsibility for submission of the necessary data. The names of those who agreed to undertake this task are shown in Appendix D, and were predominantly consultant cardiologists.

Participating hospitals were asked to submit aggregated data on the total number of PTCA procedures on a monthly basis. In addition, information was requested on any patient who died in hospital within 30 days of the procedure. If hospitals were aware of deaths occurring at home, they were invited to report these as well.

Review of deaths

For every case where NCEPOD was informed of a death within 30 days of the procedure, a questionnaire was sent to the relevant consultant cardiologist. A copy of the full questionnaire is available from NCEPOD on request. The questionnaires were identified only by a number, allocated in the NCEPOD office. Copies of procedure notes and postmortem reports were also requested. If an anaesthetist was involved in the procedure, a separate questionnaire was sent to the relevant consultant. If the patient underwent coronary artery bypass graft (CABG) surgery between PTCA and death, an additional questionnaire was sent to the consultant cardiothoracic surgeon.

Data analysis

The NCEPOD administrative staff managed the collection, recording and analysis of data. The data were aggregated to produce the tables and information in the report.

Advisory groups

The designated NCEPOD Clinical Coordinators (K Callum and K Sherry), together with the advisory group members whose names are shown at the front of this report, reviewed the completed questionnaires and the aggregated data.

Confidentiality

NCEPOD is registered with the Data Protection Registrar and abides by the Data Protection Principles. All reporting forms, questionnaires and other paper records are shredded once an individual report is ready for publication. Similarly, all patient-identifiable data are removed from the computer database.

Before review of questionnaires by the Clinical Coordinators or advisors, all identification was removed from the questionnaires and accompanying papers. The source of the information was not revealed to any of the Coordinators or advisors.

APPENDIX D - LOCAL REPORTERS

Eastern

Papworth Hospital .... Dr P M Schofield

London

Hammersmith Hospital .... Dr K J Beatt

King's College Hospital .... Dr M Thomas

London Chest Hospital .... Dr R Balcon

St George's Hospital .... Dr C W Pumphrey

St Mary's Hospital .... Ms S Smart

St Thomas' Hospital .... Dr M M Webb-Peploe

The Middlesex Hospital .... Dr R H Swanton

The Royal Free Hospital .... Dr D P Lipkin

North West

Cardiothoracic Centre, Liverpool ...... Dr R A Perry

Manchester Royal Infirmary .... Dr B Clarke

The Victoria Hospital, Blackpool .... Ms S Arthur

Wythenshawe Hospital .... Dr N H Brooks

Northern & Yorkshire

Freeman Hospital, Newcastle .... Dr S Reid

Hull Royal Infirmary .... Dr M S Norell

Leeds General Infirmary .... Mr G Tate

South Cleveland Hospital .... Dr M A de Belder

South East

Southampton General Hospital .... Dr H H Gray

The John Radcliffe Hospital ...... Dr O J M Ormerod

South West

Bristol Royal Infirmary .... Dr T Cripps

Royal Devon and Exeter Hospital .... Dr L D R Smith

Trent

Glenfield Hospital .... Ms F Stevens

Northern General Hospital .... Dr R J Bowes

Nottingham City Hospital .... Dr R A Henderson

West Midlands

Birmingham Heartlands Hospital .... Dr P F Ludman

Dudley Road Hospital .... Ms J Humphreys

Walsgrave Hospital .... Dr M F Shiu

Northern Ireland

Belfast City Hospital .... Dr G Murtagh

Royal Victoria Hospital .... Dr T Matthews

Scotland

Aberdeen Royal Infirmary .... Dr K Jennings

Glasgow Royal Infirmary .... Ms F Templeton

Royal Infirmary of Edinburgh .... Dr A D Flapan

Western General Hospital .... Dr I R Starkey

Western Infirmary .... Dr J D McArthur

Wales

Morriston Hospital .... Dr M Anderson

University Hospital of Wales .... Dr W J Penny

Independent Hospitals

BUPA Hospital Leeds .... Mr D Farrell

BUPA Hospital Leicester .... Mrs C A Jones

King Edward VII Hospital,
Midhurst .... Dr W C Brownlee

London Bridge Hospital.......................... Ms A Cleary

The Priory Hospital .... Mr J Sharp

APPENDIX E - PARTICIPANTS

Consultant cardiologists

The following consultant cardiologists returned at least one questionnaire relating to the period 1 September 1998 to 31 August 1999.

Anderson M.H.
Been M.
Bennett D.H.
Bloomfield P.
Bowes R.J.I.
Brack M.J.
Brecker S.
Buchacter M.B.
Bucknall C.
Campbell S.
Chauhan A.
Connolly D.T.
Corr L.A.
Cowie M.
Crossman D.
Cumberland D.C.
Dawkins K.
de Belder M.A.
de Bono D.P.
Fitzpatrick A.P.
Flapan A.D.
Foale R.A.
Furniss S.S.
Gibbs S.
Goode G.K.
Gray H.H.
Groves P.H.
Hall J.A.
Harcombe A.
Henderson R.A.
Howright D.R.

Jennings K.
Kennedy J.A.
Levy R.D.
Liniger N.J.
Ludman P.F.
McCoomb J.M.
Millane T.A.
Mills P.
Morgan J.
Murray R.G.
Oliver R.M.
Ormerod O.J.M.
Ramsdale D.R.
Ramsey M.W.
Reid D.S.
Roberts D.H.
Rothman M.I.
Schofield P.M.
Shahi M.
Shaw T.R.D.
Signy M.S.
Singh H.
Stewart M.
Thomas M.R.
Thomas P.
Timmis A.D.
Uren N.G.
Walker J.M.
Ward D.E.
Watson R.D.
Webb-Peploe M.M.

NCEPOD is also grateful to the small number of consultant anaesthetists and cardiothoracic surgeons who kindly completed and returned questionnaires.